My 12-Week Weight Loss Planner

Congratulations on taking one (very important) step closer to losing weight!

Thank you so much for purchasing this 12-week weight loss planner. You've made a great choice!

Keeping a close eye on what you eat, how much you move, and setting daily, weekly, monthly goals makes all the difference when it comes to losing weight and embracing a healthier lifestyle.

So please don't hide this planner in a drawer and forget about it. Pick it up, flick through the pages right now, and best of all, start writing and doodling in it.

And if you're having an off day, use it as your motivator to get back on track.

Here's to your weight loss success!

Michelle

Use your planner every day to get the best results.

Inside this 12-week weight loss planner you have space to track and record:

- a before and after picture
- your weight-loss goals (broken into smaller goals)
- Body measurements
- your plan for success
- your daily meals
- your daily water intake
- your weekly weigh-ins
- your daily steps
- your daily meal planners/meal ideas (for when you're stuck for inspiration)

Good luck! You can do this!

My 'Before' Photograph

(stick a picture of yourself, at your current weight, right here. This will help you when you need a reminder of how well you're doing.)

Measurements

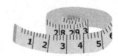

It isn't just about how much weight you lose... sometimes watching how your body is changing shape gives you a bigger boost than jumping on the scales. Use this space to write in three months' measurements – try and do this on the same day each month if possible.

Month 1:   Date:

BMI:	Waist:
Hips:	Calves:
Thighs:	Chest:

Month 2:   Date:

BMI:	Waist:
Hips:	Calves:
Thighs:	Chest:

Month 3:   Date:

BMI:	Waist:
Hips:	Calves:
Thighs:	Chest:

Plan for Success:
Month: _____

Overall Goal for the Month

Break this down into smaller goals	
1.	
2.	
3.	
4.	
5.	
6.	
7.	
8.	
9.	
10.	

Why Do You Want to Lose Weight?

Plan for Success:
Month: _____

Overall Goal for the Month

Break this down into smaller goals	
1.	
2.	
3.	
4.	
5.	
6.	
7.	
8.	
9.	
10.	

Why Do You Want to Lose Weight?

Plan for Success:
Month: _____

Overall Goal for the Month

Break this down into smaller goals	
1.	
2.	
3.	
4.	
5.	
6.	
7.	
8.	
9.	
10.	

Why Do You Want to Lose Weight?

Daily Meal Tracker

Date:

Breakfast

Snack

Lunch

Snack

Dinner

Snack

Water (tick off every glass you drink today)

Reminders

Daily Meal Tracker

Date:

Breakfast

Snack

Lunch

Snack

Dinner

Snack

Water (tick off every glass you drink today)

Reminders

Daily Meal Tracker

Date:

Breakfast

Snack

Lunch

Snack

Dinner

Snack

Water (tick off every glass you drink today)

Reminders

Daily Meal Tracker

Date:

Breakfast

Snack

Lunch

Snack

Dinner

Snack

Water (tick off every glass you drink today)

Reminders

Daily Meal Tracker

Date:

Breakfast

Snack

Lunch

Snack

Dinner

Snack

Water (tick off every glass you drink today)

Reminders

Daily Meal Tracker

Date:

Breakfast

Snack

Lunch

Snack

Dinner

Snack

Water (tick off every glass you drink today)

Reminders

Daily Meal Tracker

Date:

Breakfast

Snack

Lunch

Snack

Dinner

Snack

Water (tick off every glass you drink today)

Reminders

Daily Meal Tracker

Date:

Breakfast

Snack

Lunch

Snack

Dinner

Snack

Water (tick off every glass you drink today)

Reminders

Daily Meal Tracker

Date:

Breakfast

Snack

Lunch

Snack

Dinner

Snack

Water (tick off every glass you drink today)

Reminders

Daily Meal Tracker

Date:

Breakfast

Snack

Lunch

Snack

Dinner

Snack

Water (tick off every glass you drink today)

Reminders

Daily Meal Tracker

Date:

Breakfast

Snack

Lunch

Snack

Dinner

Snack

Water (tick off every glass you drink today)

Reminders

Daily Meal Tracker

Date:

Breakfast

Snack

Lunch

Snack

Dinner

Snack

Water (tick off every glass you drink today)

Reminders

Daily Meal Tracker

Date:

Breakfast

Snack

Lunch

Snack

Dinner

Snack

Water (tick off every glass you drink today)

Reminders

Daily Meal Tracker

Date:

Breakfast

Snack

Lunch

Snack

Dinner

Snack

Water (tick off every glass you drink today)

Reminders

Daily Meal Tracker

Date:

Breakfast

Snack

Lunch

Snack

Dinner

Snack

Water (tick off every glass you drink today)

Reminders

Daily Meal Tracker

Date:

Breakfast

Snack

Lunch

Snack

Dinner

Snack

Water (tick off every glass you drink today)

Reminders

Daily Meal Tracker

Date:
_____

Breakfast
_____

_____

Snack
_____

Lunch
_____

_____

Snack
_____

Dinner
_____

_____

Snack
_____

Water (tick off every glass you drink today)

_____

Reminders

Daily Meal Tracker

Date: _____

Breakfast
_____

_____

Snack
_____

Lunch
_____

_____

Snack
_____

Dinner
_____

_____

Snack
_____

Water (tick off every glass you drink today)

Reminders

Daily Meal Tracker

Date:

Breakfast

Snack

Lunch

Snack

Dinner

Snack

Water (tick off every glass you drink today)

Reminders

Daily Meal Tracker

Date:

Breakfast

Snack

Lunch

Snack

Dinner

Snack

Water (tick off every glass you drink today)

Reminders

Daily Meal Tracker

Date:

Breakfast

Snack

Lunch

Snack

Dinner

Snack

Water (tick off every glass you drink today)

Reminders

Daily Meal Tracker

Date:

Breakfast

Snack

Lunch

Snack

Dinner

Snack

Water (tick off every glass you drink today)

Reminders

Daily Meal Tracker

Date:

Breakfast

Snack

Lunch

Snack

Dinner

Snack

Water (tick off every glass you drink today)

Reminders

Daily Meal Tracker

Date:

Breakfast

Snack

Lunch

Snack

Dinner

Snack

Water (tick off every glass you drink today)

Reminders

Daily Meal Tracker

Date:

Breakfast

Snack

Lunch

Snack

Dinner

Snack

Water (tick off every glass you drink today)

Reminders

Daily Meal Tracker

Date:

Breakfast

Snack

Lunch

Snack

Dinner

Snack

Water (tick off every glass you drink today)

Reminders

Daily Meal Tracker

Date:

Breakfast

Snack

Lunch

Snack

Dinner

Snack

Water (tick off every glass you drink today)

Reminders

Daily Meal Tracker

Date:

Breakfast

Snack

Lunch

Snack

Dinner

Snack

Water (tick off every glass you drink today)

Reminders

Daily Meal Tracker

Date:

Breakfast

Snack

Lunch

Snack

Dinner

Snack

Water (tick off every glass you drink today)

Reminders

Daily Meal Tracker

Date:

Breakfast

Snack

Lunch

Snack

Dinner

Snack

Water (tick off every glass you drink today)

Reminders

Daily Meal Tracker

Date:

Breakfast

Snack

Lunch

Snack

Dinner

Snack

Water (tick off every glass you drink today)

Reminders

Daily Meal Tracker

Date:

Breakfast

Snack

Lunch

Snack

Dinner

Snack

Water (tick off every glass you drink today)

Reminders

Daily Meal Tracker

Date:

Breakfast

Snack

Lunch

Snack

Dinner

Snack

Water (tick off every glass you drink today)

Reminders

Daily Meal Tracker

Date:

Breakfast

Snack

Lunch

Snack

Dinner

Snack

Water (tick off every glass you drink today)

Reminders

Daily Meal Tracker

Date:

Breakfast

Snack

Lunch

Snack

Dinner

Snack

Water (tick off every glass you drink today)

Reminders

Daily Meal Tracker

Date:

Breakfast

Snack

Lunch

Snack

Dinner

Snack

Water (tick off every glass you drink today)

Reminders

Daily Meal Tracker

Date:

Breakfast

Snack

Lunch

Snack

Dinner

Snack

Water (tick off every glass you drink today)

Reminders

Daily Meal Tracker

Date:

Breakfast

Snack

Lunch

Snack

Dinner

Snack

Water (tick off every glass you drink today)

Reminders

Daily Meal Tracker

Date:

Breakfast

Snack

Lunch

Snack

Dinner

Snack

Water (tick off every glass you drink today)

Reminders

Daily Meal Tracker

Date:

Breakfast

Snack

Lunch

Snack

Dinner

Snack

Water (tick off every glass you drink today)

Reminders

Daily Meal Tracker

Date:

Breakfast

Snack

Lunch

Snack

Dinner

Snack

Water (tick off every glass you drink today)

Reminders

Daily Meal Tracker

Date:

Breakfast

Snack

Lunch

Snack

Dinner

Snack

Water (tick off every glass you drink today)

Reminders

Daily Meal Tracker

Date:

Breakfast

Snack

Lunch

Snack

Dinner

Snack

Water (tick off every glass you drink today)

Reminders

Daily Meal Tracker

Date:

Breakfast

Snack

Lunch

Snack

Dinner

Snack

Water (tick off every glass you drink today)

Reminders

Daily Meal Tracker

Date:

Breakfast

Snack

Lunch

Snack

Dinner

Snack

Water (tick off every glass you drink today)

Reminders

Daily Meal Tracker

Date:

Breakfast

Snack

Lunch

Snack

Dinner

Snack

Water (tick off every glass you drink today)

Reminders

Daily Meal Tracker

Date:

Breakfast

Snack

Lunch

Snack

Dinner

Snack

Water (tick off every glass you drink today)

Reminders

Daily Meal Tracker

Date:

Breakfast

Snack

Lunch

Snack

Dinner

Snack

Water (tick off every glass you drink today)

Reminders

Daily Meal Tracker

Date:

Breakfast

Snack

Lunch

Snack

Dinner

Snack

Water (tick off every glass you drink today)

Reminders

Daily Meal Tracker

Date:

Breakfast

Snack

Lunch

Snack

Dinner

Snack

Water (tick off every glass you drink today)

Reminders

Daily Meal Tracker

Date:

Breakfast

Snack

Lunch

Snack

Dinner

Snack

Water (tick off every glass you drink today)

Reminders

Daily Meal Tracker

Date:

Breakfast

Snack

Lunch

Snack

Dinner

Snack

Water (tick off every glass you drink today)

Reminders

Daily Meal Tracker

Date:

Breakfast

Snack

Lunch

Snack

Dinner

Snack

Water (tick off every glass you drink today)

Reminders

Daily Meal Tracker

Date:

Breakfast

Snack

Lunch

Snack

Dinner

Snack

Water (tick off every glass you drink today)

Reminders

Daily Meal Tracker

Date:

Breakfast

Snack

Lunch

Snack

Dinner

Snack

Water (tick off every glass you drink today)

Reminders

Daily Meal Tracker

Date:

Breakfast

Snack

Lunch

Snack

Dinner

Snack

Water (tick off every glass you drink today)

Reminders

Daily Meal Tracker

Date:

Breakfast

Snack

Lunch

Snack

Dinner

Snack

Water (tick off every glass you drink today)

Reminders

Daily Meal Tracker

Date:

Breakfast

Snack

Lunch

Snack

Dinner

Snack

Water (tick off every glass you drink today)

Reminders

Daily Meal Tracker

Date:

Breakfast

Snack

Lunch

Snack

Dinner

Snack

Water (tick off every glass you drink today)

Reminders

Daily Meal Tracker

Date:

Breakfast

Snack

Lunch

Snack

Dinner

Snack

Water (tick off every glass you drink today)

Reminders

Daily Meal Tracker

Date:

Breakfast

Snack

Lunch

Snack

Dinner

Snack

Water (tick off every glass you drink today)

Reminders

Daily Meal Tracker

Date:

Breakfast

Snack

Lunch

Snack

Dinner

Snack

Water (tick off every glass you drink today)

Reminders

Daily Meal Tracker

Date:

Breakfast

Snack

Lunch

Snack

Dinner

Snack

Water (tick off every glass you drink today)

Reminders

Daily Meal Tracker

Date:

Breakfast

Snack

Lunch

Snack

Dinner

Snack

Water (tick off every glass you drink today)

Reminders

Daily Meal Tracker

Date:

Breakfast

Snack

Lunch

Snack

Dinner

Snack

Water (tick off every glass you drink today)

Reminders

Daily Meal Tracker

Date:
_____

Breakfast

_____

Snack

_____

Lunch

_____

Snack

_____

Dinner

_____

Snack

_____

Water (tick off every glass you drink today)

_____

Reminders

Daily Meal Tracker

Date:

Breakfast

Snack

Lunch

Snack

Dinner

Snack

Water (tick off every glass you drink today)

Reminders

Daily Meal Tracker

Date:

Breakfast

Snack

Lunch

Snack

Dinner

Snack

Water (tick off every glass you drink today)

Reminders

Daily Meal Tracker

Date:

Breakfast

Snack

Lunch

Snack

Dinner

Snack

Water (tick off every glass you drink today)

Reminders

Daily Meal Tracker

Date:

Breakfast

Snack

Lunch

Snack

Dinner

Snack

Water (tick off every glass you drink today)

Reminders

Daily Meal Tracker

Date:

Breakfast

Snack

Lunch

Snack

Dinner

Snack

Water (tick off every glass you drink today)

Reminders

Daily Meal Tracker

Date:

Breakfast

Snack

Lunch

Snack

Dinner

Snack

Water (tick off every glass you drink today)

Reminders

Daily Meal Tracker

Date:

Breakfast

Snack

Lunch

Snack

Dinner

Snack

Water (tick off every glass you drink today)

Reminders

Daily Meal Tracker

Date:

Breakfast

Snack

Lunch

Snack

Dinner

Snack

Water (tick off every glass you drink today)

Reminders

Daily Meal Tracker

Date:

Breakfast

Snack

Lunch

Snack

Dinner

Snack

Water (tick off every glass you drink today)

Reminders

Daily Meal Tracker

Date:

Breakfast

Snack

Lunch

Snack

Dinner

Snack

Water (tick off every glass you drink today)

Reminders

Daily Meal Tracker

Date:

Breakfast

Snack

Lunch

Snack

Dinner

Snack

Water (tick off every glass you drink today)

Reminders

Daily Meal Tracker

Date:

Breakfast

Snack

Lunch

Snack

Dinner

Snack

Water (tick off every glass you drink today)

Reminders

Daily Meal Tracker

Date:

Breakfast

Snack

Lunch

Snack

Dinner

Snack

Water (tick off every glass you drink today)

Reminders

Daily Meal Tracker

Date:

Breakfast

Snack

Lunch

Snack

Dinner

Snack

Water (tick off every glass you drink today)

Reminders

Daily Meal Tracker

Date:

Breakfast

Snack

Lunch

Snack

Dinner

Snack

Water (tick off every glass you drink today)

Reminders

Daily Meal Tracker

Date:

Breakfast

Snack

Lunch

Snack

Dinner

Snack

Water (tick off every glass you drink today)

Reminders

Daily Meal Tracker

Date: _____

Breakfast

_____

Snack

_____

Lunch

_____

Snack

_____

Dinner

_____

Snack

_____

Water (tick off every glass you drink today)

Reminders

Daily Meal Tracker

Date:

Breakfast

Snack

Lunch

Snack

Dinner

Snack

Water (tick off every glass you drink today)

Reminders

Drink More Water in 30 Days

Start

Your goal...

8 glasses per day for 30 days

Water intake can help weight loss

Feeling better yet?

Keep it up... you're looking great!

You've reached your goal!

Finish

Drink More Water in 30 Days

Start

Your goal...

8 glasses per day for 30 days

Water intake can help weight loss

Feeling better yet?

Keep it up... you're looking great!

You've reached your goal!

Finish

Drink More Water in 30 Days

Start

Your goal...

8 glasses per day for 30 days

Water intake can help weight loss

Feeling better yet?

Keep it up... you're looking great!

You've reached your goal!

Finish

Weekly Weight Tracker – Weigh Yourself at the Same Time Each Week and Record it on the Scales

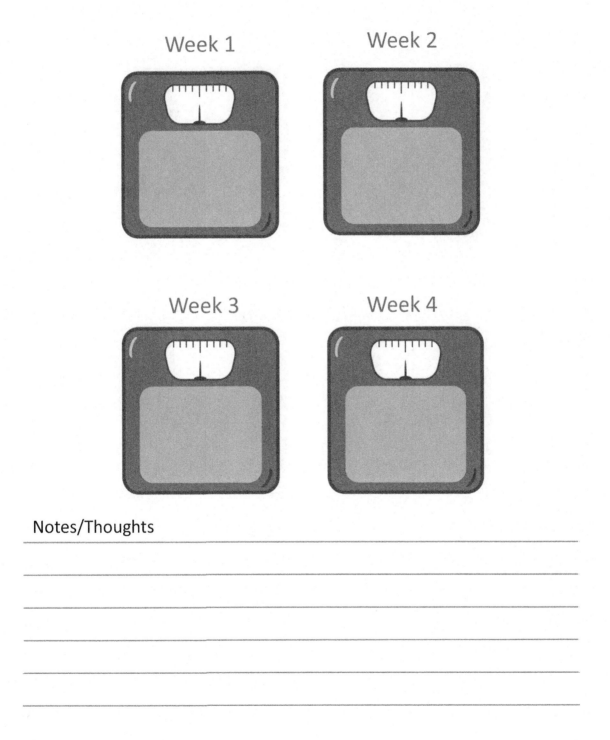

Week 1

Week 2

Week 3

Week 4

Notes/Thoughts
_____
_____
_____
_____
_____
_____

Weekly Weight Tracker – Weigh Yourself at the Same Time Each Week and Record it on the Scales

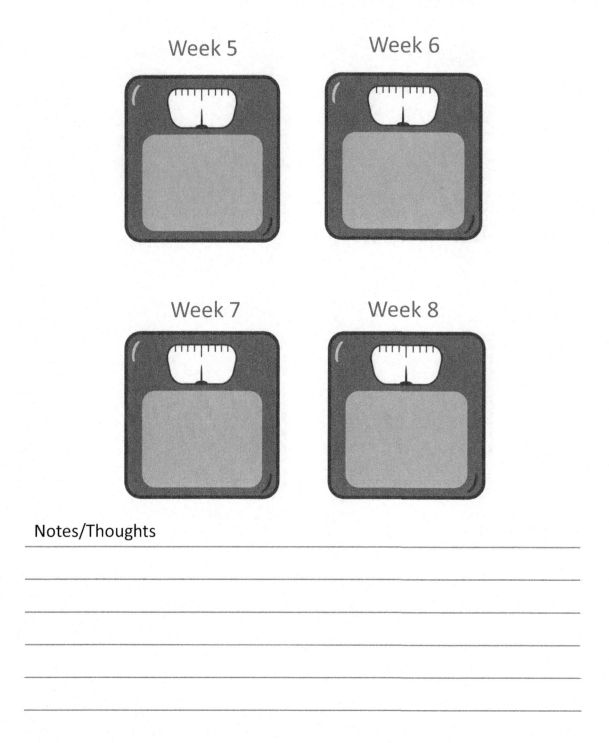

Week 5

Week 6

Week 7

Week 8

Notes/Thoughts

Weekly Weight Tracker – Weigh Yourself at the Same Time Each Week and Record it on the Scales

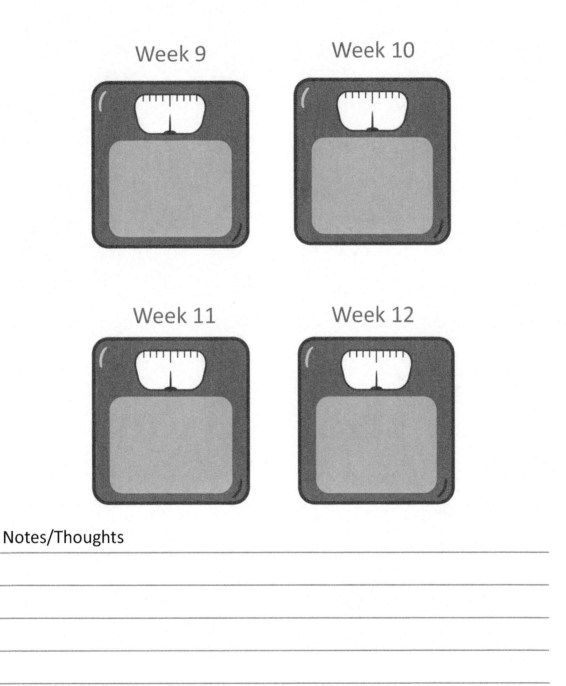

Week 9

Week 10

Week 11

Week 12

Notes/Thoughts

_____

_____

_____

_____

_____

_____

Daily Steps Tracker – How Many Steps Have you Walked This Week?

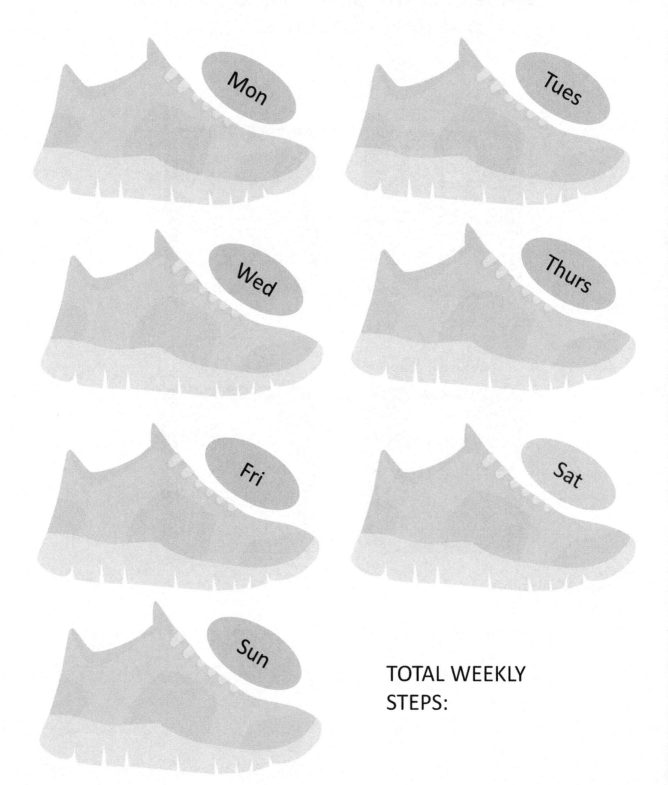

Mon

Tues

Wed

Thurs

Fri

Sat

Sun

TOTAL WEEKLY STEPS:

Daily Steps Tracker – How Many Steps Have you Walked This Week?

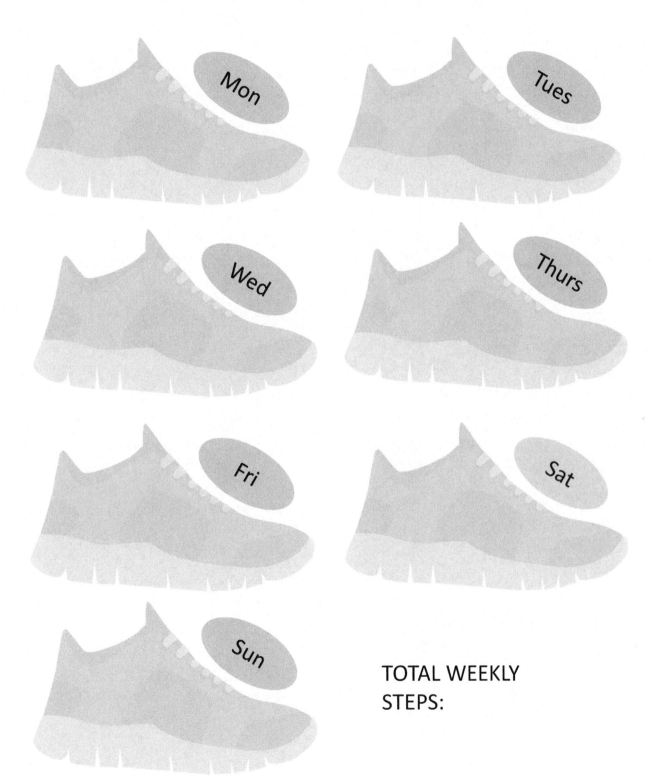

Mon

Tues

Wed

Thurs

Fri

Sat

Sun

TOTAL WEEKLY STEPS:

Daily Steps Tracker – How Many Steps Have you Walked This Week?

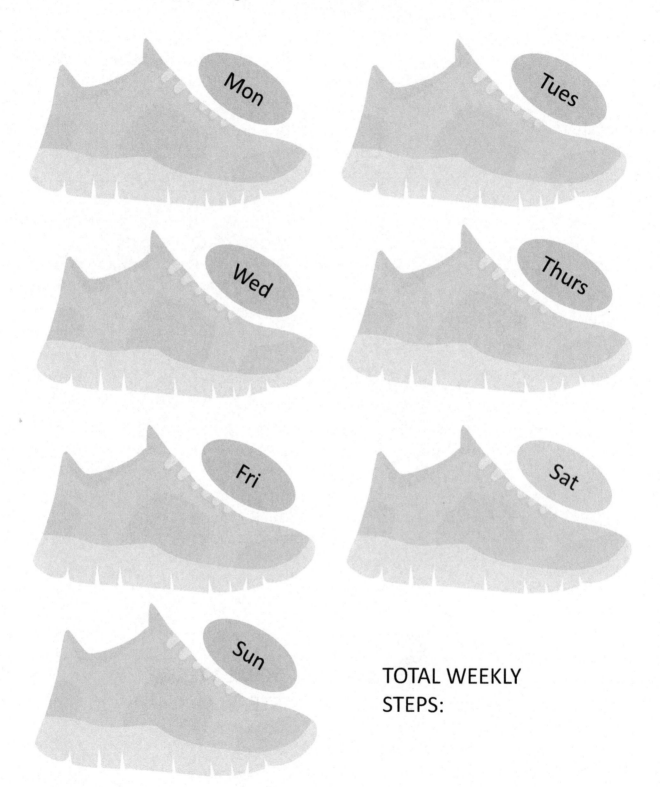

Mon

Tues

Wed

Thurs

Fri

Sat

Sun

TOTAL WEEKLY STEPS:

Daily Steps Tracker – How Many Steps Have you Walked This Week?

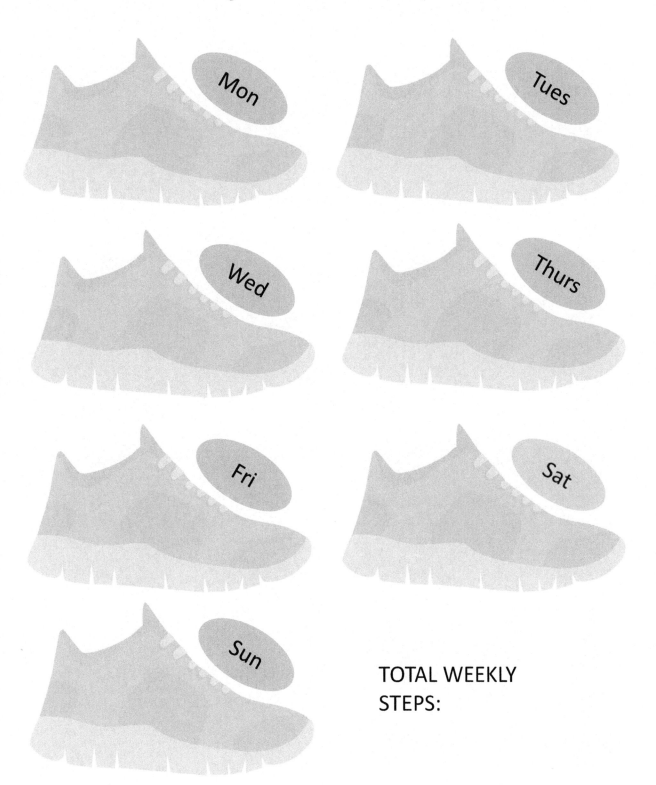

Mon

Tues

Wed

Thurs

Fri

Sat

Sun

TOTAL WEEKLY STEPS:

Daily Steps Tracker – How Many Steps Have you Walked This Week?

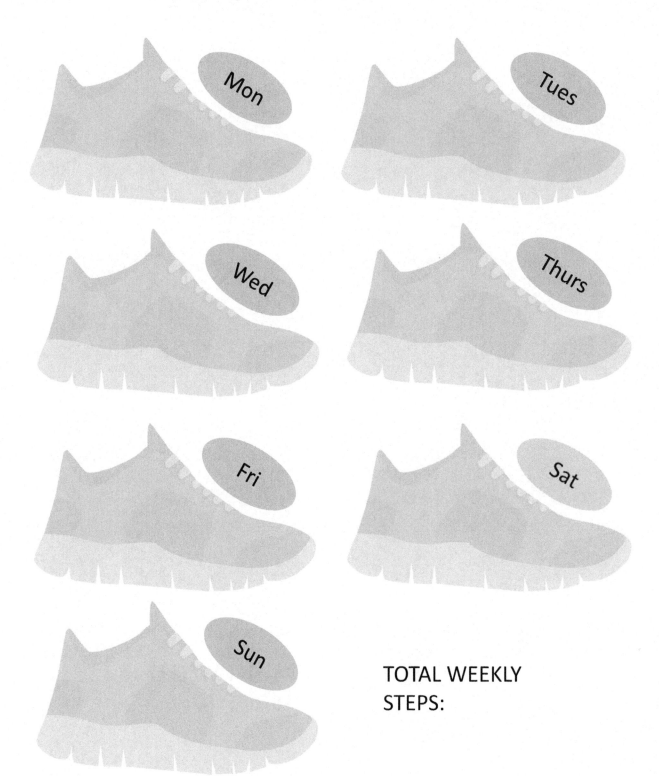

Mon

Tues

Wed

Thurs

Fri

Sat

Sun

TOTAL WEEKLY STEPS:

Daily Steps Tracker — How Many Steps Have you Walked This Week?

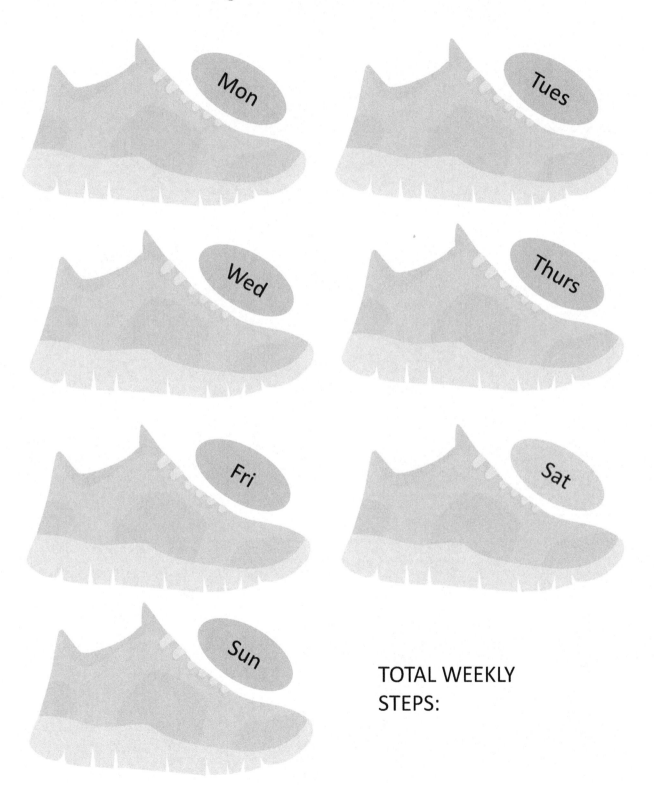

Mon

Tues

Wed

Thurs

Fri

Sat

Sun

TOTAL WEEKLY
STEPS:

Daily Steps Tracker – How Many Steps Have you Walked This Week?

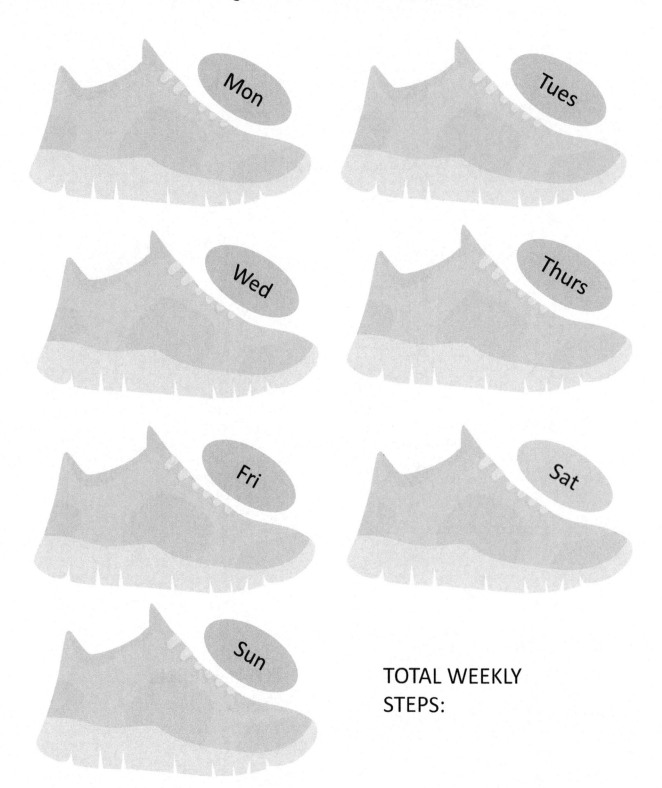

Mon

Tues

Wed

Thurs

Fri

Sat

Sun

TOTAL WEEKLY STEPS:

Daily Steps Tracker – How Many Steps Have you Walked This Week?

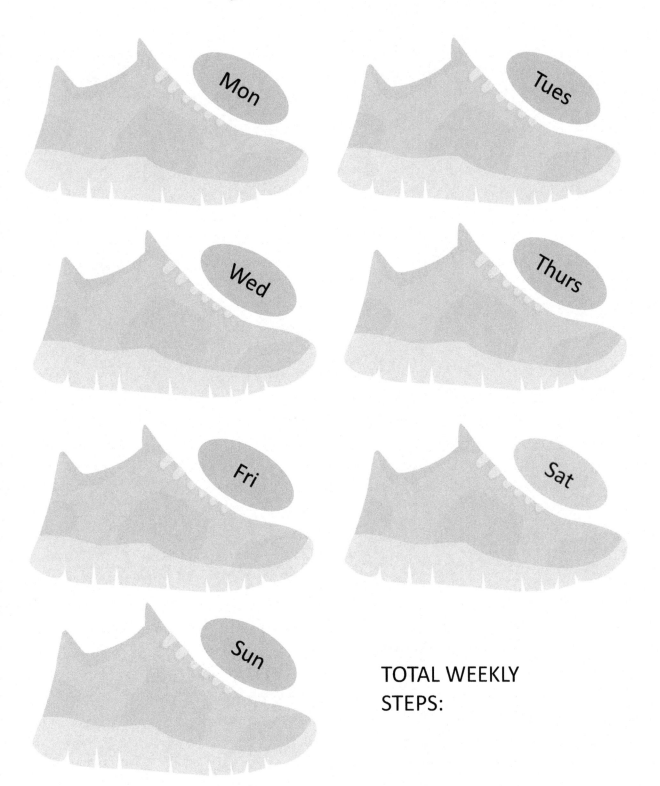

Mon

Tues

Wed

Thurs

Fri

Sat

Sun

TOTAL WEEKLY STEPS:

Daily Steps Tracker – How Many Steps Have you Walked This Week?

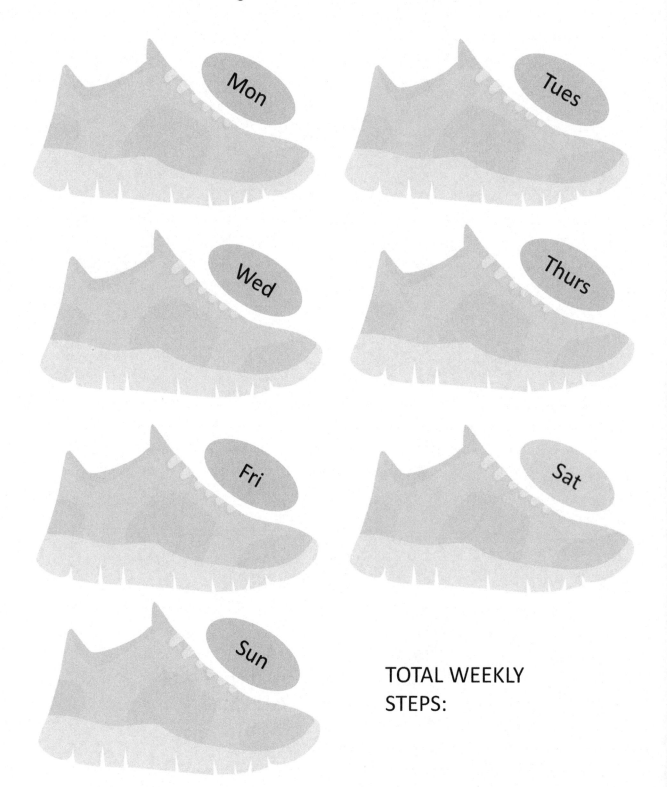

Daily Steps Tracker – How Many Steps Have you Walked This Week?

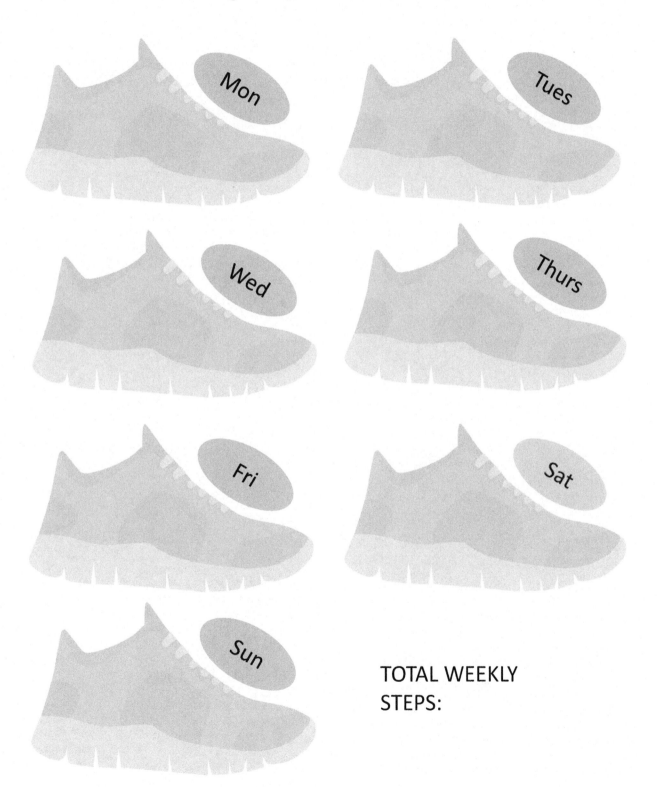

Mon

Tues

Wed

Thurs

Fri

Sat

Sun

TOTAL WEEKLY STEPS:

Daily Steps Tracker – How Many Steps Have you Walked This Week?

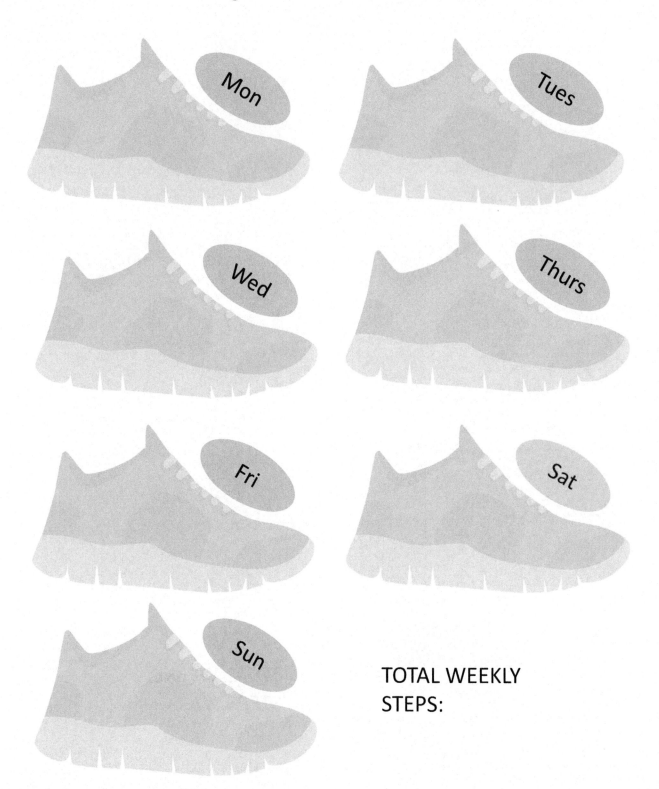

Mon

Tues

Wed

Thurs

Fri

Sat

Sun

TOTAL WEEKLY STEPS:

Daily Steps Tracker – How Many Steps Have you Walked This Week?

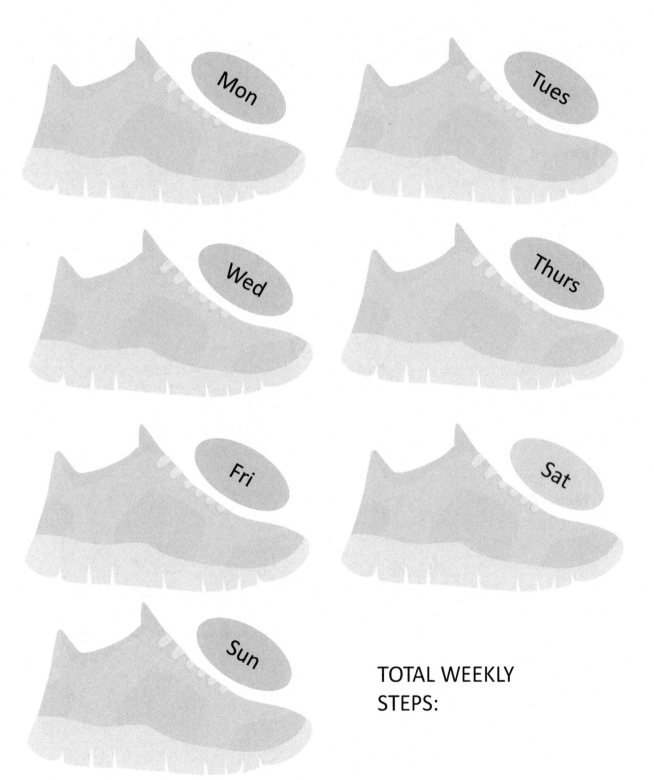

Mon

Tues

Wed

Thurs

Fri

Sat

Sun

TOTAL WEEKLY STEPS:

Meal Planner / Meal Ideas

Breakfast	
Mid Morning	
Lunch	
Afternoon	
Dinner	

Breakfast	
Mid Morning	
Lunch	
Afternoon	
Dinner	

Meal Planner / Meal Ideas

Breakfast	
Mid Morning	
Lunch	
Afternoon	
Dinner	

Breakfast	
Mid Morning	
Lunch	
Afternoon	
Dinner	

Meal Planner / Meal Ideas

Breakfast	
Mid Morning	
Lunch	
Afternoon	
Dinner	

Breakfast	
Mid Morning	
Lunch	
Afternoon	
Dinner	

Meal Planner / Meal Ideas

Breakfast	
Mid Morning	
Lunch	
Afternoon	
Dinner	

Breakfast	
Mid Morning	
Lunch	
Afternoon	
Dinner	

Meal Planner / Meal Ideas

Breakfast	
Mid Morning	
Lunch	
Afternoon	
Dinner	

Breakfast	
Mid Morning	
Lunch	
Afternoon	
Dinner	

Meal Planner / Meal Ideas

Breakfast	
Mid Morning	
Lunch	
Afternoon	
Dinner	

Breakfast	
Mid Morning	
Lunch	
Afternoon	
Dinner	

Meal Planner / Meal Ideas

Breakfast	
Mid Morning	
Lunch	
Afternoon	
Dinner	

Breakfast	
Mid Morning	
Lunch	
Afternoon	
Dinner	

Meal Planner / Meal Ideas

Breakfast	
Mid Morning	
Lunch	
Afternoon	
Dinner	

Breakfast	
Mid Morning	
Lunch	
Afternoon	
Dinner	

Meal Planner / Meal Ideas

Breakfast	
Mid Morning	
Lunch	
Afternoon	
Dinner	

Breakfast	
Mid Morning	
Lunch	
Afternoon	
Dinner	

Meal Planner / Meal Ideas

Breakfast	
Mid Morning	
Lunch	
Afternoon	
Dinner	

Breakfast	
Mid Morning	
Lunch	
Afternoon	
Dinner	

Meal Planner / Meal Ideas

Breakfast	
Mid Morning	
Lunch	
Afternoon	
Dinner	

Breakfast	
Mid Morning	
Lunch	
Afternoon	
Dinner	

Meal Planner / Meal Ideas

Breakfast	
Mid Morning	
Lunch	
Afternoon	
Dinner	

Breakfast	
Mid Morning	
Lunch	
Afternoon	
Dinner	

Meal Planner / Meal Ideas

Breakfast	
Mid Morning	
Lunch	
Afternoon	
Dinner	

Breakfast	
Mid Morning	
Lunch	
Afternoon	
Dinner	

Meal Planner / Meal Ideas

Breakfast	
Mid Morning	
Lunch	
Afternoon	
Dinner	

Breakfast	
Mid Morning	
Lunch	
Afternoon	
Dinner	

Meal Planner / Meal Ideas

Breakfast	
Mid Morning	
Lunch	
Afternoon	
Dinner	

Breakfast	
Mid Morning	
Lunch	
Afternoon	
Dinner	

Meal Planner / Meal Ideas

Breakfast	
Mid Morning	
Lunch	
Afternoon	
Dinner	

Breakfast	
Mid Morning	
Lunch	
Afternoon	
Dinner	

Meal Planner / Meal Ideas

Breakfast	
Mid Morning	
Lunch	
Afternoon	
Dinner	

Breakfast	
Mid Morning	
Lunch	
Afternoon	
Dinner	

Meal Planner / Meal Ideas

Breakfast	
Mid Morning	
Lunch	
Afternoon	
Dinner	

Breakfast	
Mid Morning	
Lunch	
Afternoon	
Dinner	

Meal Planner / Meal Ideas

Breakfast	
Mid Morning	
Lunch	
Afternoon	
Dinner	

Breakfast	
Mid Morning	
Lunch	
Afternoon	
Dinner	

Meal Planner / Meal Ideas

Breakfast	
Mid Morning	
Lunch	
Afternoon	
Dinner	

Breakfast	
Mid Morning	
Lunch	
Afternoon	
Dinner	

Meal Planner / Meal Ideas

Breakfast	
Mid Morning	
Lunch	
Afternoon	
Dinner	

Breakfast	
Mid Morning	
Lunch	
Afternoon	
Dinner	

Meal Planner / Meal Ideas

Breakfast	
Mid Morning	
Lunch	
Afternoon	
Dinner	

Breakfast	
Mid Morning	
Lunch	
Afternoon	
Dinner	

Meal Planner / Meal Ideas

Breakfast	
Mid Morning	
Lunch	
Afternoon	
Dinner	

Breakfast	
Mid Morning	
Lunch	
Afternoon	
Dinner	

Meal Planner / Meal Ideas

Breakfast	
Mid Morning	
Lunch	
Afternoon	
Dinner	

Breakfast	
Mid Morning	
Lunch	
Afternoon	
Dinner	

Meal Planner / Meal Ideas

Breakfast	
Mid Morning	
Lunch	
Afternoon	
Dinner	

Breakfast	
Mid Morning	
Lunch	
Afternoon	
Dinner	

Meal Planner / Meal Ideas

Breakfast	
Mid Morning	
Lunch	
Afternoon	
Dinner	

Breakfast	
Mid Morning	
Lunch	
Afternoon	
Dinner	

Meal Planner / Meal Ideas

Breakfast	
Mid Morning	
Lunch	
Afternoon	
Dinner	

Breakfast	
Mid Morning	
Lunch	
Afternoon	
Dinner	

Meal Planner / Meal Ideas

Breakfast	
Mid Morning	
Lunch	
Afternoon	
Dinner	

Breakfast	
Mid Morning	
Lunch	
Afternoon	
Dinner	

Meal Planner / Meal Ideas

Breakfast	
Mid Morning	
Lunch	
Afternoon	
Dinner	

Breakfast	
Mid Morning	
Lunch	
Afternoon	
Dinner	

Meal Planner / Meal Ideas

Breakfast	
Mid Morning	
Lunch	
Afternoon	
Dinner	

Breakfast	
Mid Morning	
Lunch	
Afternoon	
Dinner	

Meal Planner / Meal Ideas

Breakfast	
Mid Morning	
Lunch	
Afternoon	
Dinner	

Breakfast	
Mid Morning	
Lunch	
Afternoon	
Dinner	

Meal Planner / Meal Ideas

Breakfast	
Mid Morning	
Lunch	
Afternoon	
Dinner	

Breakfast	
Mid Morning	
Lunch	
Afternoon	
Dinner	

Meal Planner / Meal Ideas

Breakfast	
Mid Morning	
Lunch	
Afternoon	
Dinner	

Breakfast	
Mid Morning	
Lunch	
Afternoon	
Dinner	

Meal Planner / Meal Ideas

Breakfast	
Mid Morning	
Lunch	
Afternoon	
Dinner	

Breakfast	
Mid Morning	
Lunch	
Afternoon	
Dinner	

Meal Planner / Meal Ideas

Breakfast	
Mid Morning	
Lunch	
Afternoon	
Dinner	

Breakfast	
Mid Morning	
Lunch	
Afternoon	
Dinner	

Meal Planner / Meal Ideas

Breakfast	
Mid Morning	
Lunch	
Afternoon	
Dinner	

Breakfast	
Mid Morning	
Lunch	
Afternoon	
Dinner	

Meal Planner / Meal Ideas

Breakfast	
Mid Morning	
Lunch	
Afternoon	
Dinner	

Breakfast	
Mid Morning	
Lunch	
Afternoon	
Dinner	

Meal Planner / Meal Ideas

Breakfast	
Mid Morning	
Lunch	
Afternoon	
Dinner	

Breakfast	
Mid Morning	
Lunch	
Afternoon	
Dinner	

Meal Planner / Meal Ideas

Breakfast	
Mid Morning	
Lunch	
Afternoon	
Dinner	

Breakfast	
Mid Morning	
Lunch	
Afternoon	
Dinner	

Meal Planner / Meal Ideas

Breakfast	
Mid Morning	
Lunch	
Afternoon	
Dinner	

Breakfast	
Mid Morning	
Lunch	
Afternoon	
Dinner	

Meal Planner / Meal Ideas

Breakfast	
Mid Morning	
Lunch	
Afternoon	
Dinner	

Breakfast	
Mid Morning	
Lunch	
Afternoon	
Dinner	

Meal Planner / Meal Ideas

Breakfast	
Mid Morning	
Lunch	
Afternoon	
Dinner	

Breakfast	
Mid Morning	
Lunch	
Afternoon	
Dinner	

My 'After' Photo
Well done, you did it!

Printed in Great Britain
by Amazon

40374634R00086